HOMEMADE HAND SANITIZER

Practical Hand Sanitizer Recipes for a Virus-Free Lifestyle

Jailan De Luca

© Copyright 2020 by Jailan De Luca
All rights reserved.
This document is geared towards providing exact and reliable information with regards to the topic and issue covered. The publication is sold with the idea that the publisher is not required to render accounting, officially permitted, or otherwise, qualified services. If advice is necessary, legal or professional, a practiced individual in the profession should be ordered.
- From a Declaration of Principles which was accepted and approved equally by a Committee of the American Bar Association and a Committee of Publishers and Associations.
In no way is it legal to reproduce, duplicate, or transmit any part of this document in either electronic means or in printed format. Recording of this publication is strictly prohibited and any storage of this document is not allowed unless with written permission from the publisher. All rights reserved.
The information provided herein is stated to be truthful and consistent, in that any liability, in terms of inattention or otherwise, by any usage or abuse of any policies, processes, or directions contained within is the solitary and utter responsibility of the recipient reader. Under no
circumstances will any legal responsibility or blame be held against the publisher for any reparation, damages, or monetary loss due to the information herein, either directly or indirectly.
Respective authors own all copyrights not held by the publisher. The information herein is offered for informational purposes solely, and is universal as so. The presentation of the information is without contract or any type of guarantee assurance.
The trademarks that are used are without any consent, and the publication of the trademark is without permission or backing by the trademark owner. All trademarks and brands within this book are for clarifying purposes only and are the owned by the owners themselves, not affiliated with this document.

TABLE OF CONTENTS

Introduction	6
Part 1 - Basic Information	8
What is a hand sanitizer?	9
When and How to Wash Your Hands	9
Guide on the correct way to use the hand sanitizers	10
Part 2 - Recipes	11
1. Regular Homemade Hand Sanitizer	12
2. Tea Tree Oil Gel Hand Sanitizer	14
3. Essential Alcohol Hand Sanitizer	16
4. Powerful Oil Hand Sanitizer	18
5. Peppermint Gel Hand Sanitizer	20
7. Cinnamon Alcogel	22
8. Geranium Gel Hand Sanitizer	24
9. Orange Essential Oil Gel Hand Sanitizer	26
10. Tangerine Essential Oil Gel Hand Sanitizer	28
11. Sweet Orange Gel Hand Sanitizer	30
12. Lime Gel Hand Sanitizer	32
13. Myrrh Gel Hand Sanitizer	34
14. Lavender Gel Hand Sanitizer	36
15. Lemon Tee Tree Gel Hand Sanitizer	38
16. Turmeric Gel Hand Sanitizer	40
17. Bergamot Gel Hand Sanitizer	42
18. Vanilla Gel Hand Sanitizer	44
19. Lemon Spruce Hand Sanitizer	46
20. Dill Gel Hand Sanitizer	48
Conclusion	50

INTRODUCTION

In this book we are going to be talking about hand sanitizers and how the help to make you healthy especially in times of uncertainty. The use of hand sanitizers helps us protect ourselves from germs and viruses that look to infiltrate our system and make us unhealthy.

For many, the use of hand sanitizers seems to be for individuals who have a thing for staying too clean even when there is nothing to worry about. Well these viruses and diseases are real and to make us understand the importance better, we are going to be looking at some of the worst epidemics and pandemics which have ravaged the earth till date.

1. The American Plague: this happened in the 16th century, a combination of diseases which ravaged the Americans and was brought by European explorers.

2. Flu pandemic 1889-1890: this killed over 1 million people in just a few months.

3. Spanish flu 1918-1920: this killed over 100 million people.

4. Asian Flu 1957-1958: this had roots in china, killing over 1 million people.

5. Swine Flu pandemic 2009-2010: this had a high infection rate of 1.4 billion people killing around 400,000 people.

6. West African Ebola pandemic 2014-2016: about 11,000 deaths.

The truth of the matter is that hand sanitizers help us keep our hands clean, since the hand has been tagged as one of the best ways to get these viruses especially when we come in contact with them. With these hand sanitizers, you not only easily ward off anything unhealthy you come in contact with, but you also remain safe as well. We have heard time and time again about these hand sanitizers, but what exactly is it. Let us quickly define hand sanitizers before going any further.

PART 1
BASIC INFORMATION

What is a hand sanitizer?

A hand sanitizer is a liquid or gel used to reduce infectious agents which are on our hands. This alcohol-based formulation is generally more effective at killing germs and diseases on the hands and is more preferable to hand washing in antiseptic soap and water. They exist in liquid, foam, and gel formulations, something we are going to be looking at as we go further.
Simply put, hand sanitizers are healthy and we are going to be looking at how you can make then for yourself, particularly now that it is needed the most.

When and How to Wash Your Hands

Hand-washing is one of the best measures to protect yourself and your loved ones against sickness. Learn how and when your hands should be washed to be healthy.
You and your loved ones can be helped stay healthy by frequent washing of hands, especially in the most important times when germs are likely to spread and spread:
1. Before, during, and after food preparation.
2. Before food.
3. Before and after you care for a person with coughing or has diarrhea or who is sick at home.
4. Before and after a cut or wound has been treated.
5. After using the bathroom.
6. After helping a kid use the toilet or after changing the diapers or cleaning up.
7. After coughing or sneezing or after blowing your nose.
8. After feeding or taking out animal waste or even after touching

an animal.
9. After food or pet treat processing.
10. After the garbage has been touched.
11. Under a faucet, washing hands.

Every time you have to follow these five steps:
1. Wet your hands with clean, cold water, switch off the tap, and apply soap.
2. Rub them with the soap and lather your hands. Rub your fingers and under your nails. Rub your hands back and forth.
3. For at least 20 seconds, scrub your hands. Keep looking at a timer? It's almost the same as singing twice from beginning to end of a "Merry Christmas" song.
4. Use clean and running water to rinse your hands well.
5. Use a clean towel to dry your hands or dry air.

Guide on the correct way to use the hand sanitizers

When using a hand sanitizer, you have to rub it in your skin till your arms are dried. And, you're to wash your hands first with soap and water if your hands are messy or dirty.
In this context, here are some tips for the effective use of hand sanitizers:
1. Sprinkle or apply your hand sanitizer on one palm.
2. Rub your hands together thoroughly. Make sure all your hand surfaces and all fingers are covered.
3. Continue to rub for 60 seconds or till your hands are dry. For the hand sanitizer to kill more germs, it can take at least 60 seconds and sometimes even longer.

PART 2
RECIPES

Regular Homemade Hand Sanitizer

What you need:

- Measuring cup
- Measuring spoons
- Whisk
- Empty spray bottles
- 1 cup of 99% isopropyl alcohol
- 1 tablespoon of 3% hydrogen peroxide
- 1 teaspoon of 98% glycerin
- ¼ cup, 1 tablespoon, and 1 teaspoon distilled or boiled cold water

How to make it:

Step 1: Start with preparing all the things you will need.
Step 2: After that, start pouring the alcohol into a container with a pouring spout.
Step 3: Next, add the hydrogen peroxide.
Step 4: Add the glycerin and stir to combine everything.
Step 5: Then measure and pour in the water. For 99% isopropyl alcohol, measure ¼ of a cup, 1 tablespoon, and 1 teaspoon of distilled or boiled cold water and add it all to your mix then stir.
Step 6: Pour the sanitizer into the spray bottle, sanitize your spray bottles, and pour in your hand sanitizer.
That easy! You now have your hand sanitizer!

Optional for labeling:

Print or write and stick the label to the bottle.
If you don't have sticker paper, then you can print the label onto regular paper and then use clear packing tape to stick the label to the bottle by using the tape like lamination over the entire label.
Important note: squeeze or spray sanitizer generously on your hands whenever you need, or you like, then rub hands together until dry.

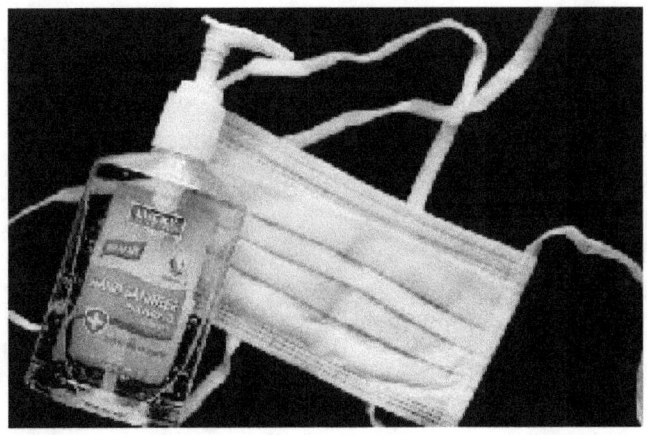

Tea Tree Oil Gel Hand Sanitizer

What you need:

- Measuring cup
- Measuring spoons
- Whisk
- Empty container bottles
- 1 cup of 91% isopropyl alcohol
- ½ cup of aloe vera gel
- 15 drops of tea tree oil

How to make it:

Step 1: Start with preparing all the things you will need.
Step 2: After that, start pouring the alcohol into a container with a pouring spout.
Step 3: After pouring the alcohol, measure and pour the aloe vera gel.
Step 4: Add the tea tree essential oil.
Step 5: Stir using a whisk to mix all ingredients.
Step 6: Pour the sanitizer into the bottle.
That easy! You now have your hand sanitizer!

Optional for labeling:

Print or write and stick the label to the bottle.
If you don't have sticker paper, then you can print the label onto regular paper and then use clear packing tape to stick the label to the bottle by using the tape like lamination over the entire label.
Important note: squeeze or spray sanitizer generously on your hands whenever you need, or you like, then rub hands together until dry.

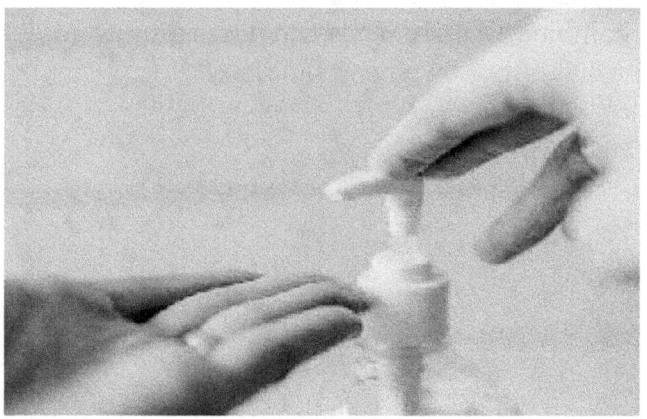

Essential Alcohol Hand Sanitizer

What you need:

- 2/3 cup rubbing alcohol h
- 1/3 cup aloe Vera
- 20 drops germ destroyer essential oil

How to make it:

Step 1: Start with preparing all the things you will need.
Step 2: After that, combine all ingredients and put in a spray bottle. That easy! You now have your own hand sanitizer!

Optional for labeling:

Print or write and stick the label to the bottle.
If you don't have sticker paper, then you can print the label onto regular paper and then use clear packing tape to stick the label to the bottle by using the tape like lamination over the entire label.
Important note: squeeze or spray sanitizer generously on your hands whenever you need, or you like, then rub hands together until dry.

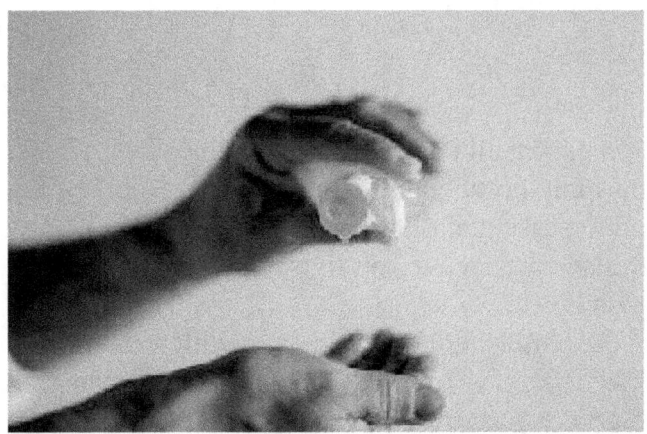

Powerful Oil Hand Sanitizer

What you need:

- 2 ounces spray bottle
- 5 drops vitamin E oil (for softer hands, this is optional)
- 2 tablespoons witch hazel with aloe vera or you can use vodka
- 5 drops of lemon essential oil
- 5 drops of orange essential oil
- 5 drops of tea tree essential oil
- Water (Distilled or at least filtered, boiled then cooled)
- Blank sticker paper for labeling (optional)

How to make it:

Step 1: Start with preparing all the things you will need.
Step 2: Then in the spray bottle, combine the vitamin E oil, witch hazel or vodka, and the essential oils.
Step 3: After that, place the sprayer on tightly and shake well for 15-20 seconds to combine.
Step 4: Next, open the bottle, and fill it to the top with water, replace sprayer, and shake again for 15- 20 seconds.
That easy! You now have your own hand sanitizer!

Optional for labeling:

Print or write and stick the label to the bottle.
If you don't have sticker paper, then you can print the label onto regular paper and then use clear packing tape to stick the label to the bottle by using the tape like lamination over the entire label.
Important note: squeeze or spray sanitizer generously on your hands whenever you need, or you like, then rub hands together until dry.

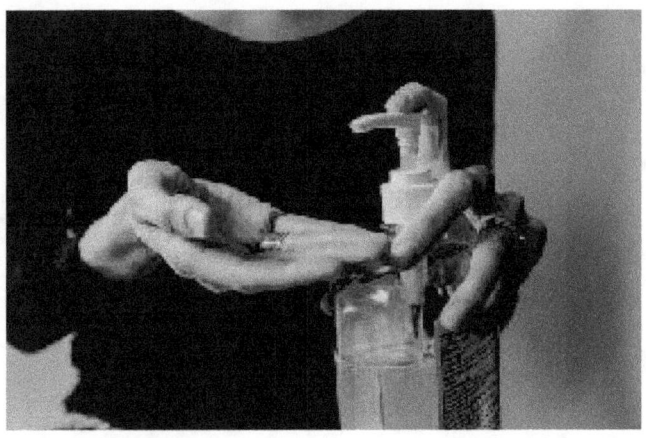

Peppermint Gel Hand Sanitizer

What you need:

- 1 small squeeze bottle
- 12 drops peppermint essential oil
- 14 drops sweet orange essential oil
- 22 drops tea tree oil
- 4 ounces aloe vera gel

How to make it:

Step 1: Start with preparing all the things you will need.
Step 2: In the small bottle, stir all the ingredients to combine correctly. That easy! You now have your own hand sanitizer!

Optional for labeling:

Print or write and stick the label to the bottle.
If you don't have sticker paper, then you can print the label onto regular paper and then use clear packing tape to stick the label to the bottle by using the tape like lamination over the entire label.
Important note: squeeze or spray sanitizer generously on your hands whenever you need, or you like, then rub hands together until dry.

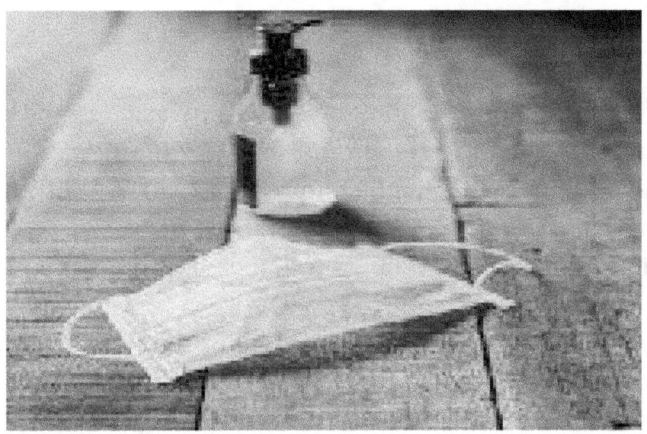

Lavender Scented Gel Hand Sanitizer

What you need:

- Bowl and spoon
- Funnel
- Bottle with a pump dispenser
- 2/3 cups of 99 % rubbing alcohol
- 1/3 cup aloe Vera gel
- 10 drops of Lavender essential oil for a pleasant scent

How to make it:

Step 1: Start with preparing all the things you will need.
Step 2: Mix all the ingredients together and then use the funnel to pour them into the bottle then screw the pump back onto the bottle.
Step 3: Make sure that the ingredients are correctly measured.
Step 4: After that, add all the ingredients together in the bowl and mix thoroughly.
Step 5: Carefully pour the mixture using a funnel into the bottle then screw the top of your bottle on tight.
That easy! You now have your own hand sanitizer!

Optional for labeling:

Print or write and stick the label to the bottle.
If you don't have sticker paper, then you can print the label onto regular paper and then use clear packing tape to stick the label to the bottle by using the tape like lamination over the entire label.
Important note: squeeze or spray sanitizer generously on your hands whenever you need, or you like, then rub hands together until dry.

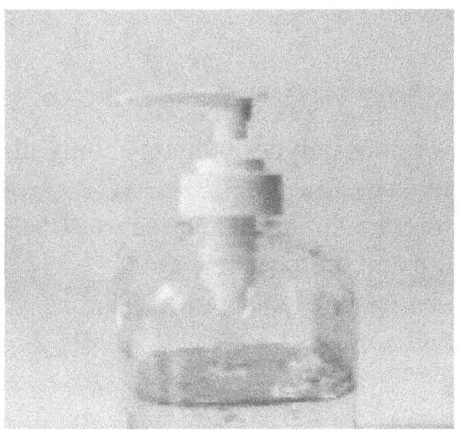

Cinnamon Alcogel

What you need:

- 1 tbsp. Rubbing alcohol
- 1/2 tsp. vegetable glycerin
- 1/4 cup aloe Vera gel
- 10 drops cinnamon essential oil
- 10 drops tea tree essential oil
- Water (Distilled or at least filtered, boiled then cooled)

How to make it:

Step 1: Start with preparing all the things you will need.
Step 2: Then mix aloe Vera gel, optional glycerin, and rubbing alcohol in a small bowl.
Step 3: After that, add the cinnamon essential oil and tea tree oil.
Step 4: Mix well and add to your desired consistency.
Step 5: After that, transfer the mixture into your bottle. That easy! You now have your own hand sanitizer!

Optional for labeling:

Print or write and stick the label to the bottle.
If you don't have sticker paper, then you can print the label onto regular paper and then use clear packing tape to stick the label to the bottle by using the tape like lamination over the entire label.
Important note: squeeze or spray sanitizer generously on your hands whenever you need, or you like, then rub hands together until dry.

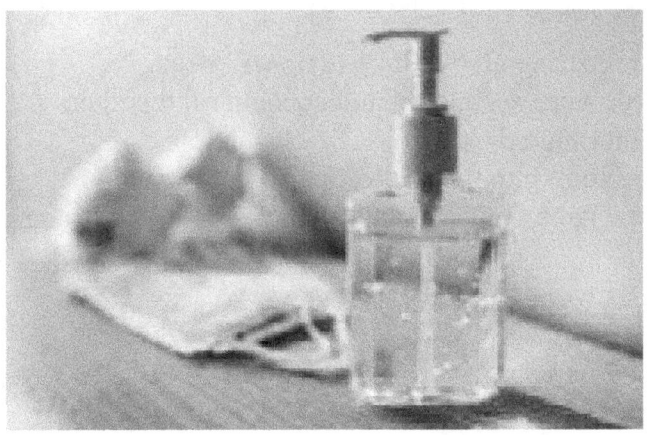

Geranium Gel Hand Sanitizer

What you need:

- 1/4 cup aloe Vera gel
- 1 tbsp. coconut oil (melted)
- 1 1/2 tbsp. witch hazel
- 5 drops geranium essential oil
- Small squeeze bottle or container

How to make it:

Step 1: Star with preparing all the things you will need.
Step 2: Mix the aloe Vera gel and melted coconut oil together.
Step 3: Add the other ingredients.
Step 4: Pour the mixture into the bottle.
That easy! You now have your own hand sanitizer!

Optional for labeling:

Print or write and stick the label to the bottle.
If you don't have sticker paper, then you can print the label onto regular paper and then use clear packing tape to stick the label to the bottle by using the tape like lamination over the entire label.
Important note: squeeze or spray sanitizer generously on your hands whenever you need, or you like, then rub hands together until dry.

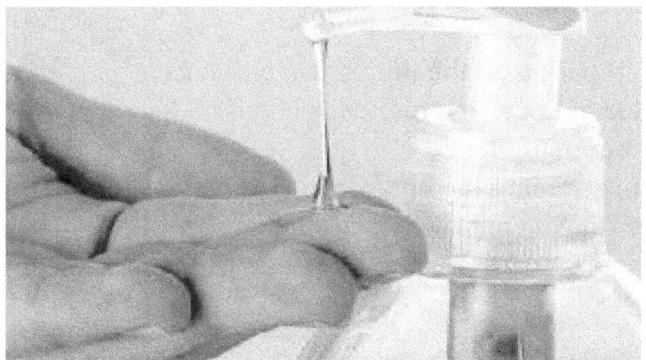

Orange Essential Oil Gel Hand Sanitizer

What you need:

- 1/4 cup aloe Vera gel
- 1 tbsp. coconut oil (melted)
- 1 1/2 tbsp. witch hazel
- 5 drops orange essential oil
- Small squeeze bottle or container

How to make it:

Step 1: Star with preparing all the things you will need.
Step 2: Mix the aloe vera gel and melted coconut oil together.
Step 3: Add the other ingredients.
Step 4: Pour the mixture into the bottle.
That easy! You now have your own hand sanitizer!

Optional for labeling:

Print or write and stick the label to the bottle.
If you don't have sticker paper, then you can print the label onto regular paper and then use clear packing tape to stick the label to the bottle by using the tape like lamination over the entire label.
Important note: squeeze or spray sanitizer generously on your hands whenever you need, or you like, then rub hands together until dry.

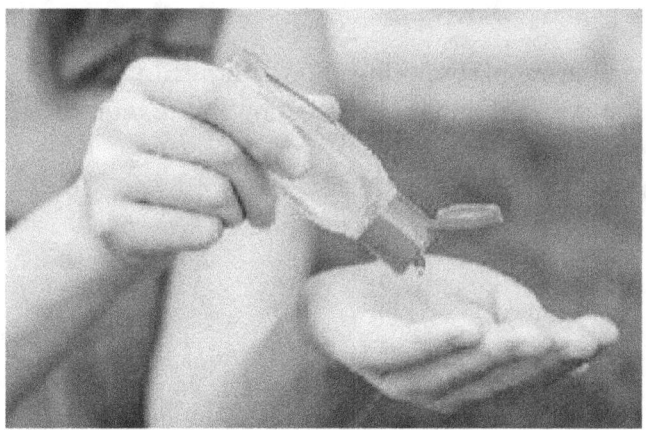

Tangerine Essential Oil Gel Hand Sanitizer

What you need:

- 1/4 cup aloe Vera gel
- 1 tbsp. coconut oil (melted)
- 1 1/2 tbsp. witch hazel
- 5 drops tangerine essential oil
- Small squeeze bottle or container

How to make it:

Step 1: Star with preparing all the things you will need.
Step 2: Mix the aloe vera gel and melted coconut oil together.
Step 3: Add the other ingredients.
Step 4: Pour the mixture into the bottle.
That easy! You now have your own hand sanitizer!

Optional for labeling:

Print or write and stick the label to the bottle.
If you don't have sticker paper, then you can print the label onto regular paper and then use clear packing tape to stick the label to the bottle by using the tape like lamination over the entire label.
Important note: squeeze or spray sanitizer generously on your hands whenever you need, or you like, then rub hands together until dry.

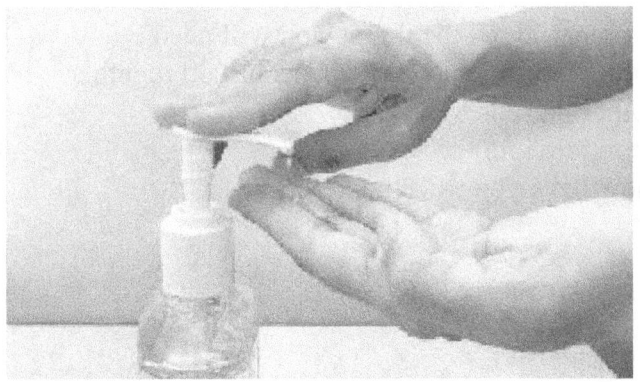

Sweet Orange Gel Hand Sanitizer

What you need:

- 1/4 cup aloe Vera gel
- 1 tbsp. coconut oil (melted)
- 1 1/2 tbsp. witch hazel
- 5 drops sweet orange essential oil
- Small squeeze bottle or container

How to make it:

Step 1: Star with preparing all the things you will need.
Step 2: Mix the aloe Vera gel and melted coconut oil together.
Step 3: Add the other ingredients.
Step 4: Pour the mixture into the bottle.
That easy! You now have your own hand sanitizer!

Optional for labeling:

Print or write and stick the label to the bottle.
If you don't have sticker paper, then you can print the label onto regular paper and then use clear packing tape to stick the label to the bottle by using the tape like lamination over the entire label.
Important note: squeeze or spray sanitizer generously on your hands whenever you need, or you like, then rub hands together until dry.

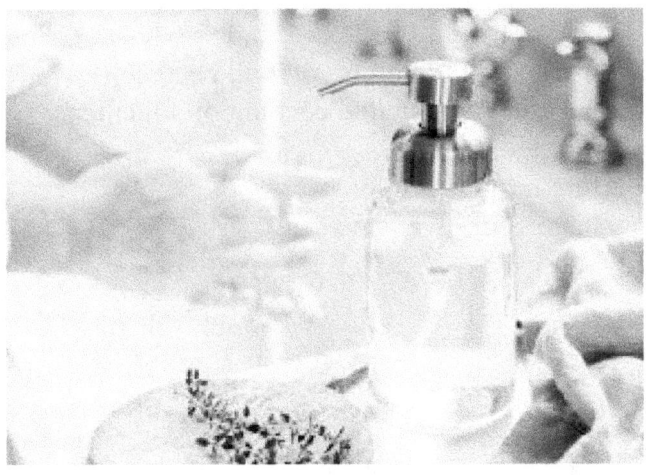

Lime Gel Hand Sanitizer

What you need:

- 1/4 cup aloe vera gel
- 1 tbsp. coconut oil (melted)
- 1 1/2 tbsp. witch hazel
- 5 drops lime essential oil
- Small squeeze bottle or container

How to make it:

Step 1: Star with preparing all the things you will need.
Step 2: Mix the aloe Vera gel and melted coconut oil together.
Step 3: Add the other ingredients.
Step 4: Pour the mixture into the bottle.
That easy! You now have your own hand sanitizer!

Optional for labeling:

Print or write and stick the label to the bottle.
If you don't have sticker paper, then you can print the label onto regular paper and then use clear packing tape to stick the label to the bottle by using the tape like lamination over the entire label.
Important note: squeeze or spray sanitizer generously on your hands whenever you need, or you like, then rub hands together until dry.

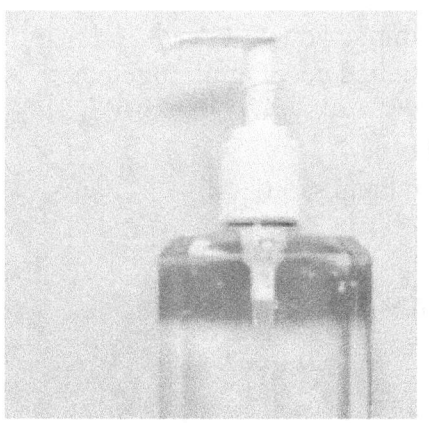

Myrrh Gel Hand Sanitizer

What you need:

- 1/4 cup aloe Vera gel
- 1 tbsp. coconut oil (melted)
- 1 1/2 tbsp. witch hazel
- 5 drops myrrh essential oil
- Small squeeze bottle or container

How to make it:

Step 1: Star with preparing all the things you will need.
Step 2: Mix the aloe vera gel and melted coconut oil together.
Step 3: Add the other ingredients.
Step 4: Pour the mixture into the bottle.
That easy! You now have your own hand sanitizer!

Optional for labeling:

Print or write and stick the label to the bottle.
If you don't have sticker paper, then you can print the label onto regular paper and then use clear packing tape to stick the label to the bottle by using the tape like lamination over the entire label.
Important note: squeeze or spray sanitizer generously on your hands whenever you need, or you like, then rub hands together until dry.

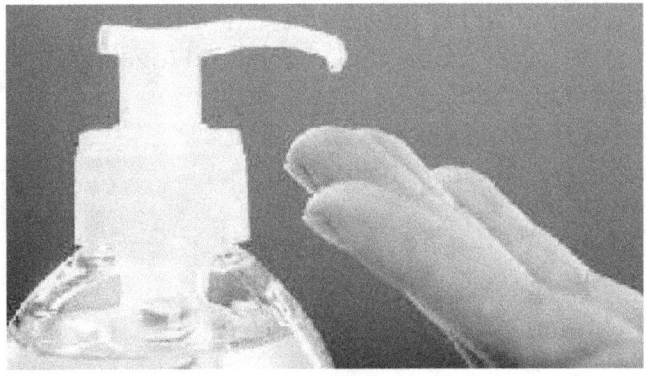

Lavender Gel Hand Sanitizer

What you need:

- 1/4 cup aloe vera gel
- 1 tbsp. coconut oil (melted)
- 1 1/2 tbsp. witch hazel
- 5 drops lavender essential oil
- Small squeeze bottle or container

How to make it:

Step 1: Star with preparing all the things you will need.
Step 2: Mix the aloe Vera gel and melted coconut oil together.
Step 3: Add the other ingredients.
Step 4: Pour the mixture into the bottle.
That easy! You now have your own hand sanitizer!

Optional for labeling:

Print or write and stick the label to the bottle.
If you don't have sticker paper, then you can print the label onto regular paper and then use clear packing tape to stick the label to the bottle by using the tape like lamination over the entire label.
Important note: squeeze or spray sanitizer generously on your hands whenever you need, or you like, then rub hands together until dry.

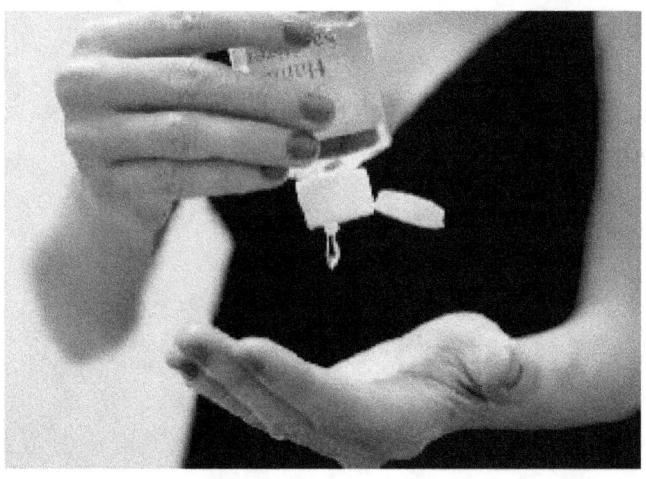

Lemon Tee Tree Gel Hand Sanitizer

What you need:

- 1/4 cup aloe Vera gel
- 1 tbsp. coconut oil (melted)
- 1 1/2 tbsp. witch hazel
- 5 drops lemon tea tree essential oil
- Small squeeze bottle or container

How to make it:

Step 1: Star with preparing all the things you will need.
Step 2: Mix the aloe vera gel and melted coconut oil together.
Step 3: Add the other ingredients.
Step 4: Pour the mixture into the bottle.
That easy! You now have your own hand sanitizer!

Optional for labeling:

Print or write and stick the label to the bottle.
If you don't have sticker paper, then you can print the label onto regular paper and then use clear packing tape to stick the label to the bottle by using the tape like lamination over the entire label.
Important note: squeeze or spray sanitizer generously on your hands whenever you need, or you like, then rub hands together until dry.

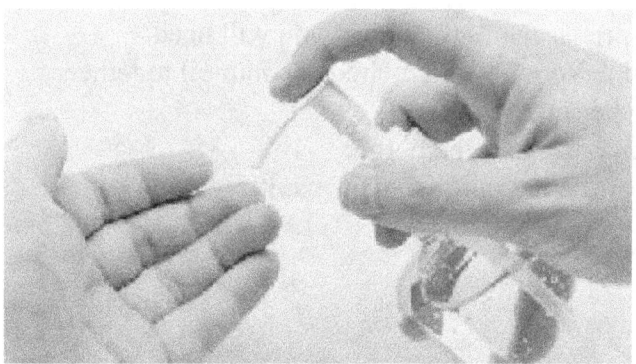

Turmeric Gel Hand Sanitizer

What you need:

- ¼ cup aloe Vera gel
- 1 tbsp. coconut oil (melted)
- 1 1/2 tbsp. witch hazel
- 5 drops turmeric essential oil
- Small squeeze bottle or container

How to make it:

Step 1: Star with preparing all the things you will need.
Step 2: Mix the aloe Vera gel and melted coconut oil together.
Step 3: Add the other ingredients.
Step 4: Pour the mixture into the bottle.
That easy! You now have your own hand sanitizer!

Optional for labeling:

Print or write and stick the label to the bottle.
If you don't have sticker paper, then you can print the label onto regular paper and then use clear packing tape to stick the label to the bottle by using the tape like lamination over the entire label.
Important note: squeeze or spray sanitizer generously on your hands whenever you need, or you like, then rub hands together until dry.

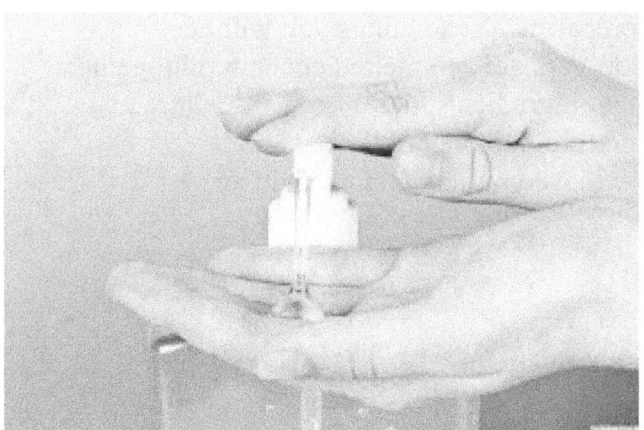

Bergamot Gel Hand Sanitizer

What you need:

- 1/4 cup aloe Vera gel
- 1 tbsp. coconut oil (melted)
- 1 1/2 tbsp. witch hazel
- 5 drops bergamot essential oil
- Small squeeze bottle or container

How to make it:

Step 1: Star with preparing all the things you will need.
Step 2: Mix the aloe Vera gel and melted coconut oil together.
Step 3: Add the other ingredients.
Step 4: Pour the mixture into the bottle.
That easy! You now have your own hand sanitizer!

Optional for labeling:

Print or write and stick the label to the bottle.
If you don't have sticker paper, then you can print the label onto regular paper and then use clear packing tape to stick the label to the bottle by using the tape like lamination over the entire label.
Important note: squeeze or spray sanitizer generously on your hands whenever you need, or you like, then rub hands together until dry.

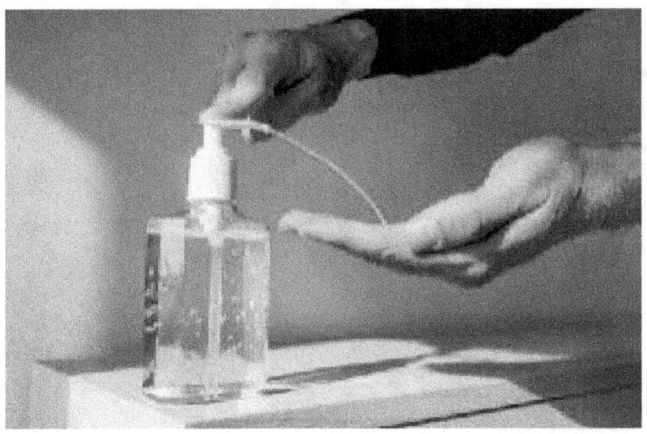

Vanilla Gel Hand Sanitizer

What you need:

- 1/4 cup aloe Vera gel
- 1 tbsp. coconut oil (melted)
- 1 1/2 tbsp. witch hazel
- 5 drops vanilla essential oil
- Small squeeze bottle or container

How to make it:

Step 1: Star with preparing all the things you will need.
Step 2: Mix the aloe Vera gel and melted coconut oil together.
Step 3: Add the other ingredients.
Step 4: Pour the mixture into the bottle.
That easy! You now have your own hand sanitizer!

Optional for labeling:

Print or write and stick the label to the bottle.
If you don't have sticker paper, then you can print the label onto regular paper and then use clear packing tape to stick the label to the bottle by using the tape like lamination over the entire label.
Important note: squeeze or spray sanitizer generously on your hands whenever you need, or you like, then rub hands together until dry.

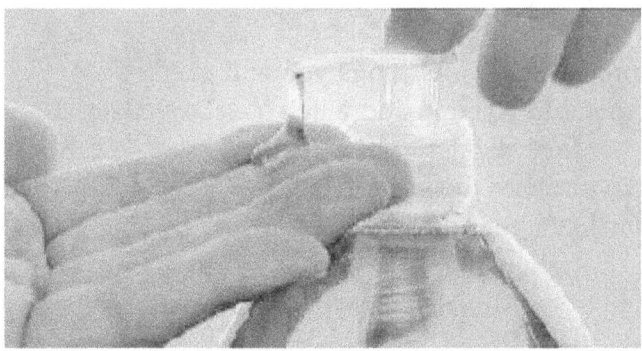

Lemon Spruce Hand Sanitizer

What you need:

- 1/2 tsp. vegetable glycerin
- 20 drops tea tree essential oil
- 10 drops spruce essential oil
- 6 drops lemon essential oil
- 3-4 tbsp. witch hazel
- Small squeeze bottle or container

How to make it:

Step 1: Star with preparing all the things you will need.
Step 2: Mix the vegetable glycerin and witch hazel together.
Step 3: Add the other ingredients.
Step 4: Pour the mixture into the bottle.
That easy! You now have your own hand sanitizer!

Optional for labeling:

Print or write and stick the label to the bottle.
If you don't have sticker paper, then you can print the label onto regular paper and then use clear packing tape to stick the label to the bottle by using the tape like lamination over the entire label.
Important note: squeeze or spray sanitizer generously on your hands whenever you need, or you like, then rub hands together until dry.

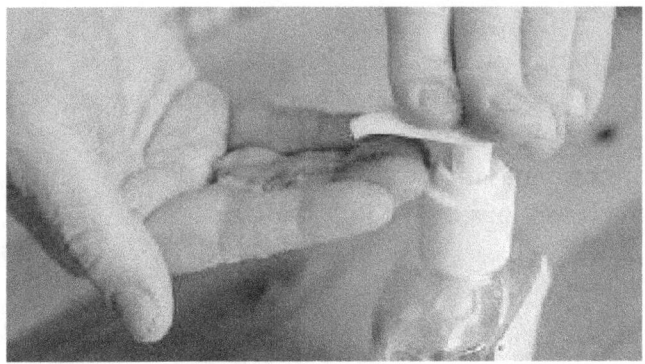

Dill Gel Hand Sanitizer

What you need:

- 1/4 cup aloe Vera gel
- 1 tbsp. coconut oil (melted)
- 1 1/2 tbsp. witch hazel
- 5 drops dill essential oil
- Small squeeze bottle or container

How to make it:

Step 1: Star with preparing all the things you will need.
Step 2: Mix the aloe Vera gel and melted coconut oil together.
Step 3: Add the other ingredients.
Step 4: Pour the mixture into the bottle.
That easy! You now have your own hand sanitizer!

Optional for labeling:

Print or write and stick the label to the bottle.
If you don't have sticker paper, then you can print the label onto regular paper and then use clear packing tape to stick the label to the bottle by using the tape like lamination over the entire label.
Important note: squeeze or spray sanitizer generously on your hands whenever you need, or you like, then rub hands together until dry.

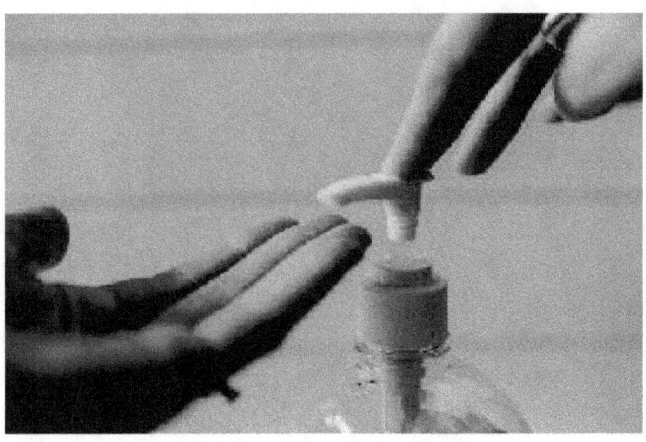

CONCLUSION

One of the most valuable assets you have is your health, and the most important thing you can do is make sure you live healthily. Hand sanitizers are scarce and expensive in times of troubles, and the best thing you can do is understand how to make them for yourself.

STAY SAFE!

www.ingramcontent.com/pod-product-compliance
Lightning Source LLC
Chambersburg PA
CBHW050312220526
45465CB00005B/1960